YOUR KNOWLEDGE HAS VALUE

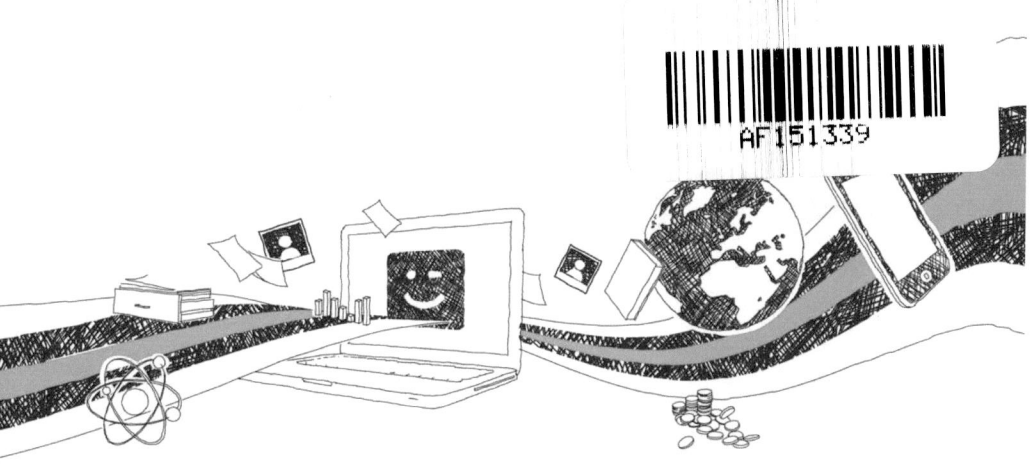

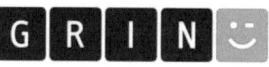

Bibliographic information published by the German National Library:

The German National Library lists this publication in the National Bibliography; detailed bibliographic data are available on the Internet at http://dnb.dnb.de .

Imprint:

Copyright © 2015 GRIN Verlag, Open Publishing GmbH
Print and binding: Books on Demand GmbH, Norderstedt Germany
ISBN: 978-3-668-03774-8

This book at GRIN:

http://www.grin.com/en/e-book/304171/a-critical-evaluation-of-the-use-of-neoni-cotinoid-insecticides-on-human

Jess White

A Critical Evaluation of the Use of Neonicotinoid Insecticides on Human Health

GRIN Publishing

GRIN - Your knowledge has value

Since its foundation in 1998, GRIN has specialized in publishing academic texts by students, college teachers and other academics as e-book and printed book. The website www.grin.com is an ideal platform for presenting term papers, final papers, scientific essays, dissertations and specialist books.

Visit us on the internet:

http://www.grin.com/

http://www.facebook.com/grincom

http://www.twitter.com/grin_com

A Critical Evaluation of the Use of Neonicotinoid Insecticides on Human Health

Insecticides are universally used, not just by farmers, but by household gardener's as a way to prevent, mitigate or repel pests. Due to outbreaks of infectious disease in honey bees and amphibians, the use of systematic insecticides has significantly increased over the last 20 years (Mason *et al.*, 2012). And is now thought to be the preferred choice; because of their toxicity and mechanistic action. One type, in particular, seen to show a usage increase is – neonicotinoids - a class of agrochemicals derived from nicotine (a substance found in cigarettes). It is thought this derivative form is solely based on the chemical similarity of the two (Calderon-Segura *et al.*, 2012). First introduced within the 1990's, neonicotinoids were principally used for their systematic nature. While most insecticides are placed on the surfaces of yielding crops, neonicotinoids are taken up by the roots and translocated to separate areas. This, therefore, makes the plant toxic to certain insect species (Pisa *et al.*, 2014). It is this mechanism of action that has now simultaneously been linked to the adverse impacts on several other invertebrate and vertebrate species (Sluijs *et al.*, 2014).

There are currently, five authorised neonicotinoid insecticides available for use in the UK, including (1) acetamiprid, (2) clothianidin, (3) imidacloprid, (4) thiacloprid, and (5) thiamethoxam (Kimura-Kuroda *et al,* 2012); these are continually divided into separate categories, known as N-nitroguanidines and N-cyano-aminides (Kanne *et al.,* 2005). Two of these insecticides, in particular, acetamiprid (ACE) and imidacloprid (IMI), are known for their cytotoxic and genotoxic effects on the human genome (Stocker *et al.,* 2004) and are currently the basis of clinical investigations among the mammalian population. Both ACE and IMI are thus, seen to have the highest adverse effects on the complete family of neonicotinoids (Stocker *et al.,* 2004).

ACE is an odourless neonicotinoid insecticide, composed of a synthetic organic compound. In insects, ACE targets the nervous system, causing paralysis and extermination, by binding to the nicotine acetylcholine receptors (nAChRs) in the neuronal pathways (Imamura *et al.*, 2010). The Environmental Protection Agency (EPA) has established that ACE is of low risk to both the environment and to human health. Risk to health can only be attributed to an adverse effect if directly contacted through consumption. ACE is, however, also a recognised irritant to human skin, which should always be handled with care in large quantities (Environmental Protection Agency, 2002). Overall, it should be noted, that ACE has been classified as an unlikely carcinogen to human health (Environmental Protection Agency, 2002).

IMI, on the other hand, is a neonicotinoid in the chloronicotinyl nitroguanidine chemical family (Horowitz *et al.*, 1998). Similar to ACE, it is widely recognised as a neurotoxin. Acting on the central nervous system (CNS), IMI blocks the nicotinergic neuronal pathway, preventing the release of the neurotransmitter acetylcholine; causing paralysis in insects (Horowitz *et al.*, 1998). Again, IMI has a low toxicity to animals and humans and has been classified as an unlikely carcinogen by EPA. IMI is, however, weakly mutagenic and must be tested for under the Endocrine Disruptor Screening Program (EDSP) (Environmental Protection Agency U.S., 2009). There is currently no published studies involving humans being chronically exposed to IMI, which has questioned as to whether IMI is toxic at all to human health. Adverse effects to IMI are completely dependent on length and level of exposure, as well as previous health records; both ACE and IMI are therefore selectively more toxic to insects than any other mammal species (Horowitz *et al.*, 1998).

In the past, both ACE and IMI have been disregarded due to their impacts on environmental ecosystems and populations. For example, the increase in neonicotinoids was found to be linked with honey bee colony collapse disorder (CCD) and a population decrease of both birds and insects (co-dependent of one another) (Gill *et al.,* 2012). It should however, be noted that the existent use for these was focused on rats and fruit flies (Yamamoto *et al.,* 1999), before there now known common use on aphids (Pesticide Action Network, 2013). Previous animal studies have indicated a low toxicity to neonicotinoids, due to the resistance of their nicotinic receptors against chemical substances. When compared to insects, however, this toxicity was increased, as protection from the blood brain barrier and central nervous system is limited (open-circulatory present) (Wu *et al.,* 2001); thus providing easy access to chemical and physical influences.

Despite the pre-misconception of neonicotinoids having a limited effect on human health, it could be argued that this class of insecticides is now thought to even play a role in the neurotoxicity of the central nervous system (CNS). Thus, the fundamental effector to adverse health effects is the human exposure to these neonicotinoids. While it may be limited, human exposure is thought to be mainly due to food and water intake. As neonicotinoids are widely used in the UK, this treatment is given to crops, during growth and before consumption; consequently increasing the attributable risk by more than 30 % (Eriksson, 1997). It is therefore thought most human exposure is self-inflicted by personal agricultural routines at home or by acquiring the produce grown in pesticide-based conditions (Mohamed *et al.,* 2009). Neonicotinoids are, however, also found in treatment creams for animals, and used to prevent or kill infestations. The residue of these neonicotinoid creams is thought to remain for up to 3-4 weeks post-usage; thus, increasing the likelihood of human contact during activities such as petting or playing (Mohamed *et al.,* 2009).

According to Kimura-Kuroda *et al.,* (2012), the reasoning behind the adverse effects from human exposure, is due to the chemical similarity of neonicotinoids and nicotine. Neonicotinoids, therefore, have the ability to share agonist (ligand-induced responses) activity at nicotinic acetylcholine receptors (nAChRs). nAChRs are the functional neuron receptor proteins that play a role in muscular contraction, upon the presence of a chemical stimulus (Purves *et al.,* 2008). It is this mechanism of action that is the key to changes within the central nervous system (CNS). As these nAChRs are cholinergic receptors, they have to ability to form ligand-gated ion channels within the plasma membrane of neurons and at the neuromuscular junction (Hibbs *et al.,* 2009). Upon the binding of acetylcholine, the ion channels open, allowing for the influx of cations, such as sodium, potassium or calcium (Gotti *et al.,* 2004); which in neuroscience is important for the regulation of signalling pathways (Stocker *et al.,* 2004). Upon the binding of a neonicotinoid, such as acetamiprid (ACE) however, it is believed this is the cause behind adverse functioning known as, developmental neurotoxicity (DNT).

In neuroscientific terms, developmental neurotoxicity is the negative change in chemical structure or function within the CNS, often caused by the presence of a chemical or physical influence. This process is often believed to occur during the neonatal development of a young child (Eriksson, 1997). Eriksson (1997) has suggested that as part of mammalian development, we have a critical period for normal maturation. He observed that a low-dosage of nicotine and nicotine-like chemicals lead to changes in adult brain function [within mice] and caused behavioural disturbances, during child development. It is thought that adult exposure to the same chemicals has a limited effect on brain function when compared to neonatal infants. Exposure at a young age is to have a long-term effect on development (Giordano *et al.,* 2012), due to increased susceptibility to neurotoxic action within the brain (Eriksson, 1997).

In a paper published by Giordano *et al.,* (2012), it was stated that for chemical / physical changes to be classed as symptoms of neurotoxicity, morphological changes including, neuronopathy (loss of neurons), axonopathy (degeneration of axons), myelinopathy (loss of glial cells) and similar gliopathies would have to present. Whether the changes were mild or temporary, prevention should be taken to reduce the exposure to infants from a neonatal age. Structural damage, whether reversible or not, will also lead to compromised function in adult life.

Grandjean *et al.*, (2006), has similarly backed-up Eriksson (1997) and Giordano *et al.*, (2012), suggesting disorders, such as autism, mental retardation and cerebral palsy are all influenced by the presence of one or more toxic chemicals during neonatal neurodevelopment. Kimura-Kuroda *et al.*, (2012) showed this through several studies, situating that in the presence of both ACE and IMI, there was an increased cellular influx of calcium (Ca2+), within the neurons; thus activating voltage-dependent calcium channels (VDCCs) and Ca2+ uptake. The preliminary uptake of Ca2+ ions by the voltage-dependent calcium channel may simultaneously act as a negative feedback signal, preventing the shift of VDCC into its non-conducting state. This in turn, suggests both ACE and IMI have the ability to pass through the blood-brain barrier, increasing the risk to human health. As these neurotoxins have a genotoxic activity, mutations of the VDC channels can arise, de-regulating Ca2+ signalling involved in synaptic formation and dendritic growth – both of which contribute to the development of autism and mental retardation (Krey *et al.*, 2007). Even with its mechanistic action, nAChR however, does have the ability to undergo desensitisation in the presence of agonist molecules, even when at low concentrations; consequently preventing any adult effects (Kimura-Kuroda *et al.*, 2012).

It should be noted that as of now, systematic testing for the influence of neonicotinoids has been prevented, due to the absence of proof. Although strong claims for its role, effects of their presence have only been tested on laboratory models (such as mice); thus, potentially suggesting that industrial chemicals like neonicotinoids may, in fact, have no effect at all (Krey *et al.*, 2007).

With regards to the lack of evidence, one study by Grandjean *et al.,* (2006) looked at pesticide exposure through the measurement of organophosphate (OPs) metabolites within children's (ages 4 and 5) urine. It was thought, pesticides chemically similar to neonicotinoids were connected with the delay in children's reaction times. Problems with short-term memory and attention span were also recorded accordingly. Those children who also showed physical development changes, were found to be born to mothers with a decreased expression level of PON1 – An enzyme required for the hydrolysis of pesticide substances (Costa *et al.,* 2005). Lowered expression of PON1, from infant exposure to neonicotinoids, has simultaneously been linked to the development of Autism in North American children (D'Amelio *et al.,* 2005). Neonicotinoids, OPs, and other pesticide-based chemicals have been seen to interfere with cholinergic signalling of the central nervous system, especially in those already with a genetic pre-disposition (Pessah *et al.,* 2008). Children displaying genetic variances in the expression of nAChR, showed a lower metabolic activity, and the reduced ability to detoxify and eliminate waste chemicals from the body. This has therefore proved to be important for environmental linked genetic studies (Pasca *et al.,* 2007).

As well as autism, Giordano *et al.,* (2012) has linked OPs to neurodegenerative diseases, such as Parkinson's or Alzheimer's; this is based on the principle of "silent damage" that establishes itself as the individual ages. Thayer *et al.,* (2012) also advocated that exposure to the use of neonicotinoids could be associated to both diabetes and obesity. Individuals who were obese, were found have elevated glucose levels when over-exposed to pesticide chemicals. Primarily this was due to the differentiation of adipocytes and / or changes in neuronal circuits that regulate eating behaviour.

Irrespective of published work to suggest neonicotinoids do play a role in affecting human health, one paper published by Tennekes *et al.,* (2013) proposes otherwise. Although pesticide chemicals can have an adverse effect on human health, the exposure would have to be high and for a long period of time to show any significant influence. Direct contact with the advocated chemical, would also increase the risk, but only if consumed at an elevated level; this was stated on the basis of adult ingestion.

To conclude, it could be proposed, that with the right care and precaution, exposure to neonicotinoids could be significantly reduced. While they are useful in the farming and veterinary industries, dependence of these should be reconsidered and replaced with natural, non-toxic alternatives. The use of neonicotinoid insecticides should also be avoided in the presence of infants, to prevent developmental neurotoxicity (DNT). As the research into this area is moderately limited, there is no significant evidence, which would suggest neonicotinoids do affect human health. Research with regards to the effects of environmental factors, does, in fact, show a strong relationship between the two; but further investigation is thus needed to confidently prove or disprove any correlation between both exposure and human health impacts.

References

BEES (2013) *Neonicotinoids.* [Online]. Available from: http://bees.pan-uk.org/neonicotinoids [Accessed: 2/11/2014].

Costa, L.G., Cole, T.B., Vitalone, A. & Furlong, C.E. (2005) Measurement of Paraoxonase (PON1) Status as a Potential Biomarker of Susceptibility to Organophosphate Toxicity. *International Journal of Clinical Chemistry.* **352**(1-2): 37-47.

D'Amelio, M., Ricci, I., Sacco, R., Liu, X., D'Agruma, L., Muscarella, L.A., ... Persico, A.M. (2005) Paraoxonase Gene Variants are Associated with Autism in North America, but Not Italy: Possible Regional Specificity in Gene-Environment interactions. *Molecular Psychiatry.* **10**(11): 1006-1016.

Environmental Protection Agency (2012) *Acetamiprid.* [Online]. Available from: http://www.epa.gov/pesticides/chem_search/reg_actions/registration/fs_PC-099050_15-Mar-02.pdf [Accessed: 2/11/2014].

Environmental Protection Agency U.S. (2009) *Endocrine Disruptor Screening Program: Tier 1 Screening Order Issuing Announcement.* [Online] Available from: http://www.epa.gov/endo/pubs/stakeholder/notices.htm [Accessed 3/11/2014].

Eriksson, P. (1997) Developmental Neurotoxicity of Environmental Agents in the Neonate. *Neurotoxicology.* **18**(3): 719-726.

Gill, R.J., Ramos-Rodriguez, O. & Raine, N.E. (2012) Combined Pesticide Exposure Severely Affects individual- and Colony-Level traits in Bees. *Nature.* **491**(7422): 105-108.

Giordano, G. & Costa, L.G. (2012) Developmental Neurotoxicity: Some Old and New Issues. *International Scholarly Research Notices.* **2012**: doi:10.5402/2012/814795 [Online Only].

Grandjean, P. & Landrigan, P.J. (2006) Developmental Neurotoxicity of Industrial Chemicals. *The Lancet*. **368**(9553): 16-22.

Hibbs, R.E., Sulzenbacher, G., Shi, J., Talley, T.T., Conrod, S., Kem, W.R., ... Bourne, Y. (2009) Structural Determinants for Interaction of Partial Agonists with Acetylcholine Binding Protein and Neuronal a7 Nicotinic Acetylcholine Receptor. *The EMBO Journal*. **28**: 3040-3051.

Horowitz, A.R., Mendelson, Z., Weintraub, P.G. & Ishaaya, I. (1998) Comparative Toxicity of Foliar and Systematic Applications of Acetamiprid and Imidacloprid Against the Cotton Whitefly, Bemisia tabaci (Hemiptera: Aleyrodidae). *Bulletin of Entomological Research*. **88**: 437-442.

Imamura, T., Yanagawa, Y., Nishikawa, K., Matsumoto, N. & Sakamoto, T. (2010) Two Cases of Acute Poisoning with Acetamiprid in Humans. *Clinical Toxicology*. **48**(8): 851-853.

Kanne, D.B., Dick, R.A., Tomizawa, M. & Casida, J.E. (2005) Neonicotinoid Nnitroguanidine Insecticide Metabolites: Synthesis and Nicotinic Receptor Potency of Guanidines, Aminoguanidines, and Their Derivatives. *Chemical Research in Toxicology*. **18**(9): 1479-1484.

Kimura-Kuroda, J., Komuta, Y., Kuroda, Y., Hayashi, M. & Kawana, H. (2012) Nicotine-Like Effects of the Neonicotinoid Insecticides Acetamiprid and Imidacloprid on Cerebellar Neurons from Neonatal Rats. *PLoS ONE*. **7**(2): e32432.

Krey, J.F. & Dolmetsch, R.E. (2007) Molecular Mechanisms of Autism: A Possible Role for $Ca^{2}+$ Signalling. *Current Opinion in Neurobiology*. **17**(1): 112-119.

Mason, R., Tennekes, H., Sanchez-Bayo, F. & Jepsen, P.U. (2012) Immune Suppression by Neonicotinoid Insecticides at the Root of Global Wildlife Decline. *Journal of Environmental Immunology and Toxicology.* **1**: 3-12.

Mohamed, F., Gawarammana, I., Robertson, T.A., Roberts, M.S., Palangasinghe, C., Zawahir, S., ... Roberts, D.M. (2009) Acute Human Slef-Poisoning with Imidacloprid Compound: A Neonicotinoid Insecticide. *PLoS ONE.* **4**(4): e5127.

Pasca, S.P., Nemes, B., Vlase, L., Gagyi, C.E., Dronca, E., Miu, A.C. & Dronca, M. (2006) High Levels of Homocysteine and Low Serum Paraoxonase 1 Arylesterase Activity in Children with Autism. *Life Science.* **78**(19): 2244-2248.

Pessah, I.N., Seegal, R.F., Lein, P.J., LaSalle, J., Yee, B.K., Van-De-Water, J. & Berman, R.F. (2008) Immunologic and Neurodevelopmental Susceptibilities of Autism. *Neurotoxicology.* **29**(3): 531-544.

Pisa, L.W., Amaral-Rogers, V., Belzunces, L.P., Bonmatin, J.M., Downs, C.A., Goulson, D., & McField, M. (2014) *Effects of Neonicotinoids and Fipronil on Non-target Invertebrates.* Berlin: Springer.

Purves, D., Augustine, G.J., Fitzpatrick, D., Hall, W.C., LaMantia, A.S., McNamara, J.O. & White, L.E. (2007) *Neuroscience.* 4th Edition. England: Sinauer Associates.

Sluijs, J.P., Amaral-Rogers, V., Belzunces, L.P., Bijleveld Van Lexmond, M.F.I.J., Bonmatin, J.M., Chagnon, M., ... Wiemers, M. (2014) Conclusions of the Worldwide Integrated Assessment on the Risk of Neonicotinoids and Fipronil to Biodiversity and Ecosystem Functioning. *Environmental Science and Pollution Research.* DOI 10.1007/s11356-014-3229-5 [Online Only].

Stocker, M., Hirzel, K., D'hoedt, D. & Pedarzani, P. (2004) Matching Molecules to Function: Neuronal Ca2+-activated K+ Channels and After-hyperpolarisations. *Toxicon: Journal of the International Society of Toxicology.* **43**(8): 933-949.

Tennekes, H.A. & Sanchez-Bayo, F. (2013) The Molecular Basis of Simple Relationships Between the Exposure Concentration and Toxic Effects with Time. *Toxicology.* **309**: 39-51.

Thayer, K.A., Heindel, J.J., Bucher, J.R. & Gallo, M.A. (2012) Role of Environmental Chemicals in Diabetes and Obesity: A National Toxicology Program Workshop Review. *Environmental Health Perspectives.* *120*(6): 779-789.

Wu, I.W., Lin, J.L. & Cheng, E.T. (2001) Acute Poisoning with the Neonicotinoid Insecticide Imidacloprid in N-Methyl Pyrrolidone. *Clinical Toxicology.* **39**(6): 617-621.

Yamamoto, I. & Casida, J.E. (1999) Nicotinoid Insecticides and the Nicotinic Acetylcholine Receptor. *Environmental Science and Pollution Research.* DOI 10.1007/s11356-014-3471-x [Online Only].

YOUR KNOWLEDGE HAS VALUE

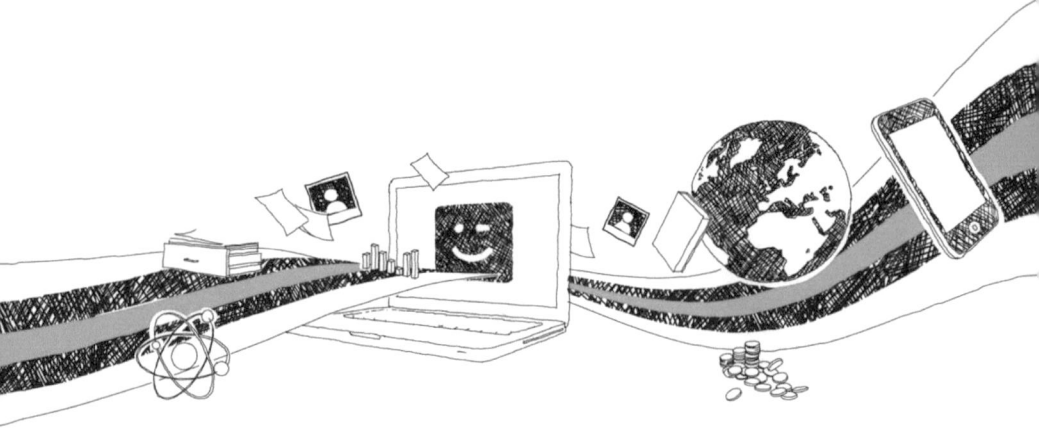

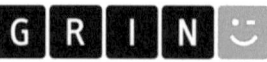